ENLARGE YOUR PENIS NATURALLY

Christopher Street

TABLE OF CONTENTS

INTRODUCTION

Hello! First, I would like to thank you for taking the time to download my eBook. I am dedicated to make sure you receive quality advice to improve your life. In this book, we will go over a wide variety of effective ways to enlarge your penis. If you are looking to increase the length or girth of your penis, then you should learn about the options that can help you meet your ambition.

The truth is, all men think about the size of their genitalia. It does not matter if you are average, above average, or even below average in terms of penile growth. I am going to be very honest with you, this book is no get big quick trick. It is not a magic lamp where a genie will pop out and grant you a wish; it is a text that will teach you the proper techniques, exercise routines, and equipment to achieve penile enlargement over a period of time. This may take several months or even years, but eventually you will be making the routine a part of daily life.

Penile enlargement training takes time and strategy. You have to know how to include it into your lifestyle. For example, fad diets are not something to try out. It has happened to many people who have tried out a trendy diet, lost 20 pounds in thirty days, but then go back and drastically gain it back the next month. Sometimes, these dieters gain more than what they originally lost! These types of diets never work because they are too difficult to incorporate into your normal life. When we all already know what works and that is eating good clean food and normal exercise on a daily basis. The person that dedicates one to two hours a day four or five days a week with a healthy diet will always be in good shape and physical fit. Jelqing in penile enlargement works in the same way with consistent stretching and exercising built into your daily life. In return, you will make small, but multiple gains consistently over time. That is if you are willing to be patient.

Besides discussing healthy eating habits and exercise, we will be learning about how hormones play a specific role in growth. You will learn about how much testosterone the average man should have. Our biology plays a big part in achieving this goal, but keep in mind that routine and motivation do too.

 I would love to tell you can gain 3 inches in a month, however, I believe in telling the pure, unadulterated truth instead of falsehoods. What I would like to help you achieve is more realistic. I can guarantee you that I can help you increase your size. Whether it is 1 ½ inches or three inches in a single year, you will definitely see and feel the difference that this program has to offer. If you are willing to put in the work and dedication, then you will meet these realistic goals.

CHAPTER 1: BASIC HEALTH AND WEIGHT LOSS

Believe it or not, your overall health is an important factor in terms of penile enlargement. You want a body that is free from any injuries or sickness that can prevent you from having the satisfaction of growing a larger penis. In order to make sure that your well-being is focused on, you must learn how to maintain your health, or improve your health if you are already out of shape. Also, let's take a look at not only our physical health, but mental health to see how both aspects can affect penile enlargement, erections, and libido.

PHYSICAL HEALTH

Physical health is a vital part of your overall well-being and fitness. In order to keep your penis healthy, you must keep your heart healthy. You see, when you are having sexual thoughts, your brain sends certain signals to your penis, making its vessels and tissues swell up with blood. In order for that to happen, your heart had to pump that blood. In order to maintain the erection and allow it to grow in size, there must be no complications with the heart or penis. If you want to make sure your blood has no problem with circulation, you have to keep your circulatory system healthy.

THE CIRCULATORY SYSTEM

The circulatory system is one of eleven systems comprised in the human body. It aids in blood and oxygen transportation, as well as hormones and nutrients to and from organs and cells. The main part of the circulatory system is the heart. Without it, your body wouldn't be able to have blood pumped. The circulatory system also aids in maintaining body temperature, sending white blood cells to fight infections, and allowing communication between hormones and organs.

EXTRA FAT, GET RID OF THAT

As said, in order to have successful penile growth and erections, the man has to keep his circulatory system healthy. Obesity can inhibit the ability to keep that system healthy, and as a result, affect the penis. You increase the risk of diabetes if you are obese, which is a condition that harms the body's circulation.

Another reason why being overweight can affect your penis is estrogen. Fat cells hold onto additional estrogen, which is a fat-storing hormone. The higher your weight, the higher your estrogen levels may become. In response, your testosterone levels lower and cause you to have trouble gaining size, erections, and libido. Energy is decreased and muscle mass lessens. You may develop what is called hidden penis, which is where a man's penis is buried underneath layers of belly fat and skin. As a man gets older, it can get increasingly worse. With knowing all of this, you can see there are many downsides in having too much fat stored in your body. Fortunately, there are things you can do to prevent it from being a huge hurdle with your growth goals

In order to increase circulation and trim fat, you will have to get active! Cardiovascular exercises such as running, walking, or cycling can train your heart and get it into shape by increasing its rate. 20 to 30 minutes a day, for five to six days a week can make a huge impact on your overall health. And you may have to buy smaller sizes in clothing.

SMOKING AND DRINKING

Smoking is something to avoid when trying to achieve penile enlargement. Not only is it a nasty habit, but affects circulation and therefore your genitals. You should be careful with those beers and shots. Too much alcohol is to be avoided since it can lead to nerve damage, shrinkage, decreased sex drive, and erectile dysfunction. This does not mean you cannot have the occasional drink once in a while. Even a glass or two of red wine can help with better circulation. Get rid of your bad habits and expect the change you have been waiting to see.

MENTAL HEALTH AND ITS IMPACT

Many men like to focus on the physical aspect of achieving length and girth to their penis, but it takes more than just physical activities and diet changes to make penile enlargement possible. Believe it or not, our mental health is as important as our physical health. Your thoughts, emotions, and behaviors are all important and are connected to your physical well-being. For example, stress can affect the brain and heart, two organs necessary for healthy genitalia for sexual intercourse.

People who feel they have inadequate penile size may feel depressed. Because of this depression, it can make working out, eating right, or even taking a shower feel like a chore. Depression can make people make bad decisions such as eating junk food, staying up late, and smoking tobacco products. Some may feel drinking a six-pack helps with feeling depressed. If you are overweight and have diabetes, you increase your chances of depression.

Anxiety has much as an impact as depression. Stress from work, school, or relationships can make you feel anxious, especially If you are someone's boyfriend or husband. Feeling overwhelmed, scared, and nervous can take a toll on heart disease, Anxiety about your penis can be harmful as it can cause uneasiness and shame. In turn, this can become an unhealthy obsession.

Whether you are depressed or anxious, be aware of the fact that there are ways around it. You have to remind yourself that you are not the only one with this issue. Many men struggle with depression and anxiety having to do with the size of their manhood. We wouldn't have the number of penile enlargement products, exercises, and diets that you see online and on television if you were the only guy! Another suggestion is relaxation exercises. Yoga and meditation are becoming even more popular in the United States. Meditation is known for helping people with pain, depression, and anxiety.

Using one or more of these solutions for the betterment of your health will take time. Mental and psychological health have to be up to par in order to succeed in your goal of a longer (or thicker) penis. Push your biological limits by solving these problems naturally.

PILLS AND FOOD

It is understandable why men wanting to gain penis size search for different brands of pills or creams to ingest or apply. Television commercials, internet advertisements, and magazines will tell the person that they guarantee 3 inches to their penis in two weeks or less. This is both financially and psychologically harmful because not only do they not work, but these companies can get your hopes up while dollars are being drained from your bank account.

Learn about the various types of pills, herbs, and foods that are commonly used to increase penis size. In this section, you will read about the truths and myths about supplementation and food in terms of penis enlargement. Hopefully, this will clear up any misinformation you may have heard of in the past.

ARE PILLS WORTH IT?

Tablets, pills, capsules: these are three common words used to describe any supplementation claiming that you will have instant penis growth on the package. While infomercials make it seem as though they work, there is no evidence showing that these supplements work. The websites that claim there are studies that show their products being successful either: (a) have no studies or (b) have studies, but contain no valid data.

Whether they are tablets, pills, or capsules, many medical professionals will agree that these are simply products that cannot enlarge your penis. The same goes for any herbs, creams, or lotions claiming the same thing. Sites marketing these pills and creams tend to not address the U.S. Food and Drug Association approval issue, which should be proof enough that they are not approved by the FDA

Eating healthy is something everyone, male or female, should be doing. When it comes to penis enlargement, there is no food that can suddenly make you grow a giant member. If you want to decrease the odds of shrinkage or dysfunction, healthy eating is great for better blood flow. You should avoid processed foods such as candy, potato chips, and chicken nuggets and replace them with fruits, homemade sweet potato chips, and baked chicken breast. Your food should contain vitamins and minerals that will keep your body energized such as:

❏ Protein

Proteins are building blocks for the body. It is known for building strong muscles, bones, skin, nails, and hair. Additionally, protein helps with enzyme and hormonal production, which is good for males to keep their genitalia as well as the rest of the body's tissues, healthy and functional. On average, adults need about 40 to 65 grams of protein. Foods such as eggs, beef, and chicken breast have protein. The best way to calculate how much you need is by taking how much you weigh in pounds and convert it to kilograms. Next, multiply by 0.8 kilograms. A sedentary male needs about 56 grams per day.

❏ Complex Carbohydrates

If you are looking for more energy, complex carbohydrates will do the trick. Complex carbohydrates are made of multiple sugar molecules known as polysaccharides that are linked in a chain instead of only one or two sugar molecules in simple carbohydrates (known as monosaccharides). Complex carbs are rich in fiber and help with overall health. They are mainly found in plant foods, so you will definitely receive tons of minerals and vitamins. Men need at least 38 grams of fiber and 50% to 60% of a person's diet should consist of carbohydrates.

❏ Lycopene

Lycopene is an antioxidant that can lower the chance of heart disease and cancers such as prostate cancer. This can aid in infertility and help with aging. Even though some people do not consider lycopene as an "essential mineral," it is still suggested to include in your diet. Men should take 9 mg per day. Foods such as tomatoes and berries are lycopene-laden fruits that can improve your health in the long run. If you cannot eat tomatoes, look into fresh watermelon.

❏ Omega 3 Fatty Acids

Omega 3 Fatty Acids are essential nutrients for overall body health such as blood clotting and protection against heart disease and certain cancers. Men would most definitely benefit from these essential nutrients since they aid with circulation so that arteries are able to pump blood to the penis for long, hard erections. Keep in mind there are different types of fatty acids from various food sources such as fish and green vegetables like broccoli or kale. Multivitamins or fish oil capsules will contain omega 3 fatty acids if you are not looking to eat your way to a healthy hard-on.

❏ Zinc

Many of you may have heard of health benefits zinc delivers for men. If you have ever bought a multivitamin, or compared a men's multivitamin to a women's multivitamin, you will notice that there is more of this mineral in the men's. Zinc is a metal that is known as an essential trace element. In other words, even though it is a metal, it is a metal that is good for you in minute amounts. Men need at least 11 milligrams daily. One of the advantages of taking zinc is the increased libido and testosterone levels. It also allows sperm to be healthy and keep moving in numbers. So, if you want to have children in the future, you will want zinc to strengthen and accelerate your sperm's speed.

❏ Vitamins A, C, and E

You have always heard as a kid you need to take your vitamins so you can get big and strong. Well, even as a grown man, vitamins are great at helping you get "big and strong." Vitamins A, C, and E are the trio you want in your corner against the fight of inadequate penile size and impotency.

-Vitamin A is perfect for reproduction purposes keeping your penis healthy, and eschewing infection. You need a strong immune system, so vitamin A will do the trick.

-Vitamin C is necessary for overall development and growth. Healthy skin, bones, and muscles need vitamin C. It is one of those vitamins that you definitely need to keep taking since it expelled through urination very easily.

-Last, but not least, vitamin E is a fat soluble vitamin that works on body circulation and repairs tissues. Adults need about 15 milligrams each day.

CHAPTER 2: THE ANATOMY OF THE PENIS

If you have taken sex education or have read biology or medical texts, you will see physical structures of male and female genitalia. Diagrams, short descriptions, and labels are a few things you may have seen as you were imbibing all of this information. Heck, over the years, you have heard different names for your penis. Peter, Johnson, and dick were (and still are) commonly used when referring to a man's parts. As you are searching for answers about what can be used or done to increase the size of your penis, it is important to learn about the science and the structure of the penis in detail. If you have never learned in-depth about the penis's structure, I suggest you do so before using the natural alternatives shown in the following chapters.

FUNCTION OF THE PENIS AND STARTING WITH A TIP

Besides sexual function, the purpose of the penis is to expel urine. That opening that allows semen and urine to exit is called the meatus. It is the external part of the urethra. The head (or mushroom-like) part of the penis is known as the glans. On the glans, is an area called the mucosa. The mucosa is a tissue that is covered over the glans to keep it moist. Next, the glans and mucosa is covered by a skin sheath called the prepuce, or foreskin. The foreskin is very important for many reasons including lubrication for the glans, aid for penetration during intercourse, and reduce chafing and friction. Many parents may choose to have their son's foreskin removed for religious or traditional reasons. As a result, the mucosa that was once moist develops into dry skin. After the glans, is the corona. It is the rigid tissue that connects the glans to the length of the penis.

THE TISSUE TRIAD

Now, let's get into the types of erectile tissue that make up the penis. The shaft, which is the length of the penis between the glans and the scrotum, is made up of three tissues. First, the corpus cavernosum. This is comprised of two tissues that run along the sides of the penis. When you have an erection, these tissues are filled up with blood to make your penis expand and rise. The second type of tissue, which is the third tissue, is called the corpus spongiosum. This is the tissue that runs down the frontal part of the penis, down towards the glans while still allowing your urethra to be open.

CHAPTER 3: HOW HORMONES AFFECT PENIS GROWTH

Hormones play a significant role in the advancement of penis enlargement. Hormones are chemical substances in the body that are responsible in the regulation and control of cells and organs. In science courses from high school and college, as well as discussions about puberty, you may have heard of two key hormones: testosterone and estrogen. These hormones are pretty complex when it comes to penile development and overall male puberty. Too much or too less of something can have significant consequences. Learn about these two hormones and how they contribute to the enlargement of a man's penis and sex drive.

WHAT IS TESTOSTERONE?

You may have heard of phrases such as "high testosterone" or "low testosterone" at the doctor's office or during normal conversation, especially when referring to males. Testosterone is a steroid hormone that can be found in a biological male's testes. It can be found in a biological female's ovaries as well, but in very small amounts in comparison to males. Testosterone is a hormone in the androgen group that is responsible for primary and secondary male characteristics. It is a force that is responsible for reproduction, increased muscle mass, increased body hair, and a deeper, coarser voice. Since the sex organs (penis, testes) are primary male characteristics, testosterone affects both the growth of the penis as well as the libido.

You see, when a man can get his hormone levels measured with a test known as a serum total testosterone test. Testosterone is present and is divided into two categories: bound testosterone and free testosterone. It is measured by nanograms per deciliter (ng/dl). Keep in mind that the men's testosterone levels are between 270 ng/dl and 1070 ng/dl, with the average levels being 679 ng/dl.

HOW DHT AFFECTS PENIS LENGTH AND GIRTH

Penis development is based on the presence and amount of dihydrotestosterone (DHT). DHT is a sex steroid and androgen hormone that comes from testosterone. Free testosterone acts as a prohormone, and with the aid of the 5alpha reductase enzyme, breaks down into this type of androgen hormone that aids in the growth of one's penis. Without DHT, enlargement cannot be achieved because it is with DHT that androgen receptors can respond in the shaft of the penis.

As a man ages, his testosterone levels will decline. This can happen during the 30s and 40s, but can also occur while a man is in his 20s. Because of age and testosterone reduction, it can change the appearance, size, curvature, and sensitivity. Be aware that this does not apply to all men. As said before, a man in his 20s can have low testosterone levels, resulting in penile enlargement and libido issues while someone three times his age can have average testosterone levels with no issues present.

Usually, men ages 30 and older will start to see changes in their bodies, especially with their genitalia. Appearance is a big concern for many men. The glans, which is the head of the penis, will start to lose its purple hue. In addition to this, public hair will start to thin out. This is caused by the lack of blood flow and the decrease in testosterone levels. When hormone levels change, so can weight. If a man gains weight, the penis will look smaller in size.

Signs of low testosterone do not simply end at penile changes or a reduced sex drive. Soft or shrunken testes, constant hot flashes, loss of muscle mass, irritability and depression can follow. It can be devastating facing these issues, especially if you are a young man. Thankfully, you can find out what is causing it and what can be done to help.

MEDICAL CAUSES OF LOW TESTOSTERONE

A medical condition can cause low testosterone levels. Hormonal disorders, type 2 diabetes, testicular injuries, and liver and/or kidney disease are just a few examples than can inhibit proper hormonal distribution. Be sure to speak with a medical professional before looking into more natural options to increase hormonal production.

WHAT IS ESTROGEN AND WHAT IS ITS ROLE?

Estrogen is a steroid hormone that is found in women, but can be found in small trace amounts in men. When a man has too much or too little testosterone, estrogen will increase, causing difficulty in achieving penile growth. For example, an obese man may have more estrogen in his system because his fat cells contain estrogen. This can affect hormonal levels.

Too much testosterone, especially if a man chooses to increase his levels in an unnatural way, causes aromatization. Aromatization is the conversion of excess testosterone to estrogen, which is caused by an enzyme known as aromatase. This is something to avoid as men can have issues with enlargement as well as erection. Estrogen, in large amounts, is not something I would advise on having, correct levels are necessary to help keep your body health and functioning.

HOW CAN WE DETERMINE IF A MAN CAN GROW?

While it is possible for grown men to achieve length and girth to his penis, there are a few factors that come into play that must be looked at. Age and DHT levels are very important to consider whether or not enlargement can occur. Although it is impossible to change one's age, we can increase hormone levels naturally. Genetics and medical conditions have to be considered as well. With proper options such as a change in diet or exercise, you can improve those odds.

WHAT CAN BE DONE

Weight management, proper diet chock full of vitamins and minerals, and certain physical activities can aid in increasing the width and length of up to 1 or 2 inches. You have to boost your hormonal levels to get to where you are having growth. Do not feel discouraged as there are plenty of options that can be used to increase your testosterone levels naturally. If you are willing to change your life around, you will meet your goals without a problem.

CHAPTER 4: JELQING AND HOW TO WARM UP

Now that you have learned more about the importance of health and how different systems of the body come into play, now it is time to learn the proper exercises you need in order to make your penis grow. Jelqing is defined as exercising the penis to increase its length and girth. Jelqing, also known as "milking," is a physical therapy technique using circulation and blood pressure to increase the size of a man's member. The history is believed to have begun in the Middle East around 400 B.C., when fathers would teach their sons how to massage the member to make it grow larger. Others believe the term "jelq" was created by college students and simply spread across the globe.

Men from all walks of life use jelqing to strengthen and broaden their size, all while practicing safety procedures and taking their time. Before any jelqing exercise, you must warm up and prepare yourself prior to exercising. This is similar to how warm-ups are suggested before lifting weights, for example.

HOW TO WARM UP

Warming up is very simple, but many men decide to skip this step. They may feel as though warming up is unnecessary and takes away from the actual workout. This isn't true. It is suggested to warm up before any exercise to avoid any sprains, rips, tears, or discolorations. Who would want nerve damage to happen? A minimum of ten minutes is all it takes to get your penis prepared before a workout.

1.) Dip a small cloth or towel in hot water. Make sure it fully soaked and then squeeze any excess water.
2.) Carefully massage the penis. You want to make it aroused and erect half-way. This can be achieved in the shower with soap and water, but can be done outside of the shower, too.
3.) Once aroused, wrap and cover the penis with the hot cloth or towel. Make sure the glans and shaft are covered completely.
4.) Do 10 to 15 kegels* with the towel wrapping the penis. This will increase blood flow and open up the capillaries (small blood vessels located in the tissues).
5.) Take the towel or cloth off and dry off your penis. You are now prepared for your first exercise.

*Kegels are exercises for the pelvic floor muscles to improve urination and sexual function. Men simply contract the muscles behind the base of the penis, which will cause the base to rise towards the abdomen and the testicles to rise upwards.

CHAPTER 5: LENGTH EXERCISES

If you are a man looking to lengthen your penis, then you should try any of these penile length exercises. Remember: use the proper "OK" grip to avoid injury.

A-Stretch

This penile lengthening exercise is medium intensity and has a medium-level risk of injury. The A-Stretch penis enlargement exercise starts by taking your left hand and grabbing the head of the penis, pulling slightly upward and forward until you reach your comfortable stretching limit. The shaft of the penis is over your right wrist and your right hand is open, facing downward. The purpose of this exercise is to stretch the top section of the shaft, thus making it larger.

2. Basic Stretch

If you are looking for a low intensity, low-level injury risk exercise, try out the Basic Stretch. The Basic Stretch is considered the "bread and butter" of penile length exercises. Not only is length increased, but you are able to target the areas in angles. Begin by taking your right hand and placing it on the top of the penis. Next, pull the penis up forward for a comfy upwards pull. Afterwards, pull the penis to right and hold. Next, use your left hand and pull forward by the head. Lastly, pull the penis to the left and hold.

3. Double Rotation Stretch

This is high-intensity with medium risk of injury. Retract the foreskin of the penis and grab the penis with your right hand. Pull forward and around like a circle (360 degrees). Make sure you make an "OK" sign with your other hand and grab part of the shaft that is closest to your body.

4. Double Stretch

This is a simple, low-risk, and medium intensity exercise, the Double Stretch starts with one hand pulling the penis forward from behind the glans. The other hand is placed around the just above the base closest to your body, using an "OK" sign grip. Both hands pull in opposite directions.

5. Gentle Stretch

If you want to use a low intensity, low-risk exercise, try out the gentle stretch. First, take your left hand and place it behind the glans. Next, gently pull the penis forward and hold for the rep. The point is to hold the penis for a few seconds and release. It is perfect when you are on your bathroom break at school or work.

6. Hot Kegel Stretch

Add a few inches to your pecker with this exercise. Easy to do, first start off by getting your penis to erection level, wrap a hot wrap around it, and retract any foreskin. After retraction, grab your penis from behind the glans (head) and slowly pull forward. Hold the stretch and clench your pubococcygeus muscle, or PC muscle. Hold for the rep and slowly release the PC muscle, but still hold the stretch with your hand.

7. Internal Stretch

This stretch will help stretch out the part of the penis that is hidden internally away from the body. It is best to sit down with your legs wide open for this exercise. Grip the base of the penis (like an "OK" sign) and around the scrotum.

Pull penis and scrotum upwards towards the body. With the second hand, grab the penis from behind the glans and pull upwards. Relax after each rep.

8. Rotation Stretch

Here is another length enlargement exercise that is very similar to the double rotation stretch. The rotation stretch starts with the penis at erection level. Grab the penis with the ok-grip from behind the glans. Make sure the foreskin is retracted first. Next, pull the penis upward slowly until you meet your comfort limit. While still stretching your penis upwards, rotate it. If you are using your left hand, rotate to the right and vice versa. When you are rotating halfway (your glans facing down), pull the penis downward. A full circle is one repetition.

9. Twisted Stretch

The twisted stretch is an easy exercise where you stretch and twist the penis. First, make sure the penis is at erection level. Next, use both hands to twist the shaft of the penis. Grasp the penis just before the glans and pull forwards until you meet you limit. Hold it for a few seconds and release; this is considered one rep.

10. V-Stretch

V-stretch beings with the penis being partially erect. Grasp the penis just below the head and pull forward. Next, take the thumb of your second hand (while still pulling with the first hand) and place it halfway on the shaft. Press the thumb downwards gently. Repeat this as you move your thumb to different points of the shaft.

With practice and starting with low reps, you can increase the level of intensity starting from simple exercises to the more challenging ones. Now that you know how to target the length aspect of penile enlargement, you should learn about to "broaden the staff," so to speak.

CHAPTER 6: GIRTH EXERCISES

Increase the width of your penis by performing these ritualistic exercises. Remember the proper set-up prior to starting any one of these exercises.

1. Clamping

Clamping involves using a clamp instrument, allowing a limited amount of blood to flow into the penis. First, have your penis at the proper erection level, and wrap your penis with a piece of cloth or rubber such as a sock. Next, place clamp over the wrapped material. Make sure the clamp is closest to your pubic bone.

Close the clamp loosely on the base of the penis. Get yourself aroused enough to get your penis as erect as possible. Push the clamp against the pubic bone and tighten it, without creating any discomfort or pain. Keep the clamp on and do Kegel exercises to cause blood flow into the penis, while timing yourself. After time limit for the rep is over, or have feelings of pain and discomfort, stop the exercise as soon as possible and apply a hot wrap around the penis for five minutes.

It is suggested to rest in between sets. After resting, repeat by clamping like before and continuing from there. After you are done with the final set of the clamping exercise, remove the wrap around your penis.

2. Double Erect Squeeze

If you want a bigger upper shaft and glans (also called "head"), then the double erect squeeze will make you pleased. Simply get your penis to the suggested erection level. Next, grip around the base as close to you as possible using the standard or overhand ok-grip. Afterwards, do the same grip you did at the base of the penis, only grab underneath the glans. Make sure the grip of both hands are tight, then hold for that repetition. Lastly, release until you are ready for the next rep.

3. Double Squeeze

Remember reading about the corpus cavernosum? It is the tissue on the side of the penis. Since there are two of these types of tissues, they are called corpora cavernosa, located at the sides of the penis in the shaft. Blood will be forced into this area as well as the glans. The double squeeze, or double static squeeze, begins with bringing the penis to a "mid-erection". Using the ok-grip, grasp the penis at the base as close to you as possible. Right in front of the first hand, do an overhand ok-grip. Tighten the grip and the fingers on the shaft. Hold and release grips for the repetition. Between sets, you may alternate hands.

4. Dry Jelq

Expansion of cell walls is intended here to bring more amounts of blood into the shaft. One of the fundamental girth-increasing exercises, the Dry Jelq begins with the penis brought to the suggested erection level. At the middle of the shaft, grip with a loose ok grip. Next, pull the skin on the shaft back with the ok grip towards the base of the penis, getting close to the pubic bone. Slowly, slide the ok grip upwards towards the back of the glans with enough pressure. If it's too uncomfortable, use less pressure but still enough to allow blood flow.

5. Erect Squeeze

Also called ULI, the Erect Squeeze increases the size of the glans and upper area of the shaft. Blood from the lower area of the shaft is shifted upwards to the beginning part of the penis. First, bring the penis to the suggested level of erection. Second, at the base of the penis, create a standard or reverse ok grip. Squeeze as tight as possible and increase the number of fingers of the grip as necessary. Hold this position for the time length suggested and release. For the next rep, repeat the grip from before and squeeze. Between sets, be sure to switch hands.

6. Flaccid Bend

The Flaccid Bend is one of the fundamental exercises used to widen the penis. Two hands will be utilized for this exercise. First, make sure to bring your penis at the level of erection suggested. Next, with the reverse ok grip, slowly pull the penis forward until you are at a comfortable stretch. Take your second hand and place two fingers underneath the penis. Continue to stretch as you take the penis and bend it over the fingers of the second hand. Hold for the count.

Afterwards, repeat the act but instead of the two fingers being underneath the penis, press these fingers on the left or right side of the penis. You can place the fingers above the penis for an upward bend. Stretch and bend the penis onto fingers.

7. Side Jelq

There are many variations of the jelq. The Side Jelq primarily focuses on the sides and curve of the penis. The penis enlargement exercise starts by applying a lubricant to the hands as well as the penis. Be sure that the penis is at the level of erection suggested for a better outcome and experience. Use a standard ok grip around the base of the penis. Make sure it is as close to the pelvic bone as possible. Tighten the grip and slowly shift upwards, halfway up the shaft. The goal is to force blood upwards to the top of the penis, so apply as much pressure as needed.

Take the second hand and hold the penis at the base for support. Keep stroking upwards like before as you turn the penis to the side, pushing the shaft against the second hand. As you are moving upwards, reaching just before the glans, release the grip and take the palm of your first hand to stroke the penis upwards in the same direction. When the palm of your hand reaches the gland, this counts as one rep. With this exercise, you will switch hands and sides (curve penis to the left for the left side, and vice versa).

8. Vertical Jelq

This is an easy, low injury-risk exercise used to straighten a penis's upward curve. Lubricant is first added to the hands as well as the penis. Once the penis is at the suggested erection level, make a standard ok grip at the base of the penis, as close to the pubic bone as possible.

 Next, tighten the base grip and slowly move upwards on the shaft. Stop halfway on the shaft while simultaneously applying pressure to the base grip for blood flow. For support, take your second hand and grip at the base. Keep stroking upwards with the first hand will curving the penis downwards and bending the shaft over the second hand.

Discontinue once the first hand is up to the head of the penis. This is one repetition; remember to switch hands and repeat the same movement for the next repetition.

9. Wet Jelq

Another easy, low intensity penile enlargement exercise is known as the Wet Jelq. The Wet Jelq pushes blood to the two on the sides of the penis. Although it is mostly for width, this exercise has been reported to increase length as well.

First, apply lubricant to penis and hands, then bring penis to suggested erection level. At the base of the penis, make an ok grip (standard or overhand) as close to the pubic bone as possible. Tighten grip and slowly move upwards on the shaft towards the glans. Apply enough pressure as you squeeze the grip for the repetition. Stop the hand right before it reaches the glans.

Hold the grip. Take your second hand and use the standard or overhand ok grip on the base of the penis. Repeat the same move as done before for the next repetition.

CHAPTER 7: SHAPE EXERCISES

Create the perfect shape for your penis to make it more aesthetically-pleasing and make insertion easier and more pleasurable. Each exercise is low intensity and has low risk of injury.

1. Edging

If you are looking for the fundamental exercise that aids with penile enlargement and works on improved shape, then edging will do the job. As one of the best enhancement exercises, edging is when certain areas of the penis are triggered via stimulation, and before ejaculation, stimulation is stopped. After the feeling of ejaculation disappears, the person rubs those trigger areas all over again.

The first thing the man does is apply lubrication to the penis and hands. Once the penis is erect, you have to massage the base and up towards the glans. Next, go further up to massage the glans. Once you are feeling as though you are about to ejaculate, you have to slow down and move back towards the base of the penis. Stroking should be discontinued once feeling as though you're about to ejaculate (cum). This means if you were to continue to stroke, this will cause ejaculation.

Take deep, slow breaths and wait until the urge of ejaculation stops. Wait a few seconds and then go back and stroke for the rest of the exercise. Back and forth, you will be stroking until you feel as though you have to ejaculate, but then controlling those urges by stopping the strokes and taking deep, slow breaths. After finishing the exercise, you may continue stroking until you ejaculate. When you are more experienced, you can learn to stop the urges of ejaculation by doing a reverse kegel exercises for control.

2. Erect Raise

The Erect Raise is a great exercise because of its ability to make the pelvic muscle stronger. First, make sure your penis is fully erect for this exercise. Next, kegel (contract) your pelvic muscle. While holding the kegel, place your hand above the penis. Slowly push the penis downward while still holding and tightening the kegel clench. Hold it for the repetition. After the rep, slowly release the push of your hand to allow the penis to rise back up again. Lastly, release the kegel clench. This aids in blood circulation, ejaculation control, and the overall shape of the penis.

3. Helicopter Shake

While this exercise has a funny name, the Helicopter Shake is very useful in your goal of improved penile enlargement and shape. First, have your penis erect approximately half-way (40% to 50%). Next, using the standard ok grip, grip the base of your penis with your dominant hand. The dominant hand should be the hand you write with. Make sure the grip is as close to the pubic bone as possible. After you secure the grip, make circular movements with your wrist, causing the penis to rotate. Increase the rotation speed until you can make five rotations per second. Keep doing it for the duration of the exercise. Between each rep, change directions.

4. Hot Kegel Clench

The Hot Kegel Clench works on erection strength, shape, and overall circulation. In order to have a healthy penis, you also need to have healthy pelvic muscles, so this should be done regularly. It is used for warm-ups before performing other exercises. Begin with a slight erection, not 100% erect, but definitely more than halfway. Take a hot wrap and place it around the shaft. Hold the penis horizontally and clench your pelvic muscle. Hold it for the repetition. Release the pelvic muscle. For more reps, repeat by clenching the pelvic muscle and holding it before releasing it again.

5. Hot Wrap

This exercise is very simple, with only three steps to follow. Hot Wrap should be used prior to any major penile enlargement exercises. Before any workout, you must make sure the penis is warmed up. A warmed up penis allows more elasticity and better effects from the stretches (jelqing). Besides targeting the shape of your penis, you will notice how it helps against injuries. First, bring an erection that is about halfway. Next, wrap a hot wrap* around the shaft. Then, hold the wrapped shaft in your hand for the repetition. Make sure to reheat the wrap when it gets lukewarm.

*Note: Make sure you have a heated wrap in hand. You can place a heating pad in the microwave or soaking a small towel in hot water and reheating when necessary. Best temperatures to use range between 104° and 113° F (40° and 45° C).

6. Kegel Clench

The Kegel Clench builds strength to the pelvic floor muscles. In order to have a well-functioning member, the pelvic muscles must be in top condition. Not only will the penile shape improve, but you can gain multiple orgasms while keeping your prostate healthy and in shape. After bringing the penis to a full erection, clench the pelvic muscle and hold it for the repetition. Release the pelvic muscle and repeat the clench for a number of reps.

7. Towel Raise

Bring the penis to full erection and place a towel on the penis. This will act as a weight. Breathe in slowly and kegel (clench pelvic muscle) to lift the towel as high up as possible. Hold the kegel for the suggested time. Next, slowly breathe out and release the kegel to allow the penis to go back down. This is considered one repetition.

If the erection doesn't stay in place, you may place one or two fingers under the shaft to finish the set. You can also change the weight of the towel by switching towels or wetting the towel for extra weight.

CHAPTER 8: CLAMPS AND CLAMPING

During your research on penile enlargement, you may have come across the familiar term "clamp" or "clamping." Although mentioned before as one of the exercises in the girth section, it is helpful to go in-depth as to what clamping is truly about. Clamping is a penis enlargement exercise that involves a device called a clamp. The clamp restricts blow flow out of the penis while containing blood flow into the penis in a limited amount. As a result, pressure builds, and expands the tissues within the penis for increased growth whenever the man has an erection. Multiple repetitions of clamping will help this expansion become more permanent.

No newcomers to penis enlargement exercises should clamp. Clamping should only be done after six months of penile enlargement exercises and training, so practice the other exercises before doing this one. Caution and awareness is needed when utilizing clamps. Do note that the difficulty level of clamping is medium, but the intensity and injury of risk is high. You have to have an erection level of 90 % to 100%, so a full erection is necessary for this exercise.

How to Begin:

1. First, bring the penis to the suggested erection level, which is a full erection.
2. Next, wrap the base of the penis with a piece of rubber, cloth, or first aid wrap. Some people use a long piece of an old mousepad, stocking, or sock.
3. Put the clamp instrument over the wrapped base as close to the pubic bone as possible. Make sure the clamp is placed loosely when it's closed.
4. Make sure the penis is stimulated to get as erect as possible. Push the clamp against the pubic bone and get it as tight as possible without causing pain or discomfort.
5. During the rep, keep the clamp on and perform Kegel exercises so that blood presses inside the penis. Keep the full erection.
6. Release the clamp once you finish timing the repetition, or when you feel discomfort, tingling, or pain. Discontinue the exercise and apply a hot wrap around the penis for five minutes.
7. Rest in between sets to allow blood to circulate the penis and relax the erection. When ready, repeat from step 3 until all sets are completed.
8. After completing the final set, remove the fabric wrap from step 2.

Since clamping focuses mainly on girth, you will notice after numerous times of exercising that your glans (or head) is thicker when it erect or flaccid. The same can be said about the shaft. If you want to make sure you are getting the timing accurate, use the timer from your phone, computer, microwave, or even an egg timer. As for the clamp, you can buy one that is made specifically for penile enlargement online, or find a reusable cable clamp at a store. Hose clamps have been used, but they are more circular and the penis is more triangular (dorsal) internally, so it can be more difficult to remove from the penis after usage. Find what works best for you.

CHAPTER 9: PENIS PUMPS

As I'm sure you have heard in your search for various products created specifically to increase the length and girth of a man's penis, you will have come across another device known to do just that: the penis pump. A penis pump is a cylinder-shaped device with a pump that literally lets you pump up the size of your penis, both in length and girth. There is a huge variety of pumps and they may be manually operated (by hand), automatically operated (battery-powered), or hydraulically powered.

The most conventional penis pump on the market, the vacuum hand pump, which can be bought in a typical adult store, works with a fairly simple mechanism. The man fits an airtight cylinder over the penis which creates a partial vacuum around it. Using a lubricant helps create an airtight seal around the penis, it may also be necessary to shave pubic hair to avoid breaking the seal. The blood and fluid in your penis will try to move to the lower pressure air created in the vacuum which then engorges the erectile tissue more than it can typically become engorged.

There are three main uses here, the first is just to give you a temporarily firmer erection, and you can remove the vacuum after a short session and then go on to have sex, some reports indicate that the effects can last for one or two days. The second is for sexual enjoyment, many find that the sucking sensation a pump creates is very enjoyable and it's perfectly possible to achieve orgasm when using it. Lastly, the idea is to use the pump regularly to try and stretch and train the tissue of the penis so that it is slightly larger and so that you can achieve firmer and bigger erections when you want to have sex (which is typically the main goal of penis enlargement anyway).

To try and use the pump to best effect you need to have regular pumping sessions. You place the pump carefully around your penis and then provide it with slow and regular pumps while trying to maintain an erection. You can do this with different types of sexual stimulus or by trying to masturbate without ejaculation (commonly called edging). If you attempt this for 10 – 20 minutes a few times a week you should see some permanent improvement in your penis size and erectile strength. Some beginners find that their penis looks a little distorted after the first few times they use a pump: this is mostly a mind trick and it should return to its normal appearance by the next day.

You cannot speed the process up by pumping intensely early on, anymore than working out incredibly intensely will help you build muscles quicker. You want to work with a lower pressure over a longer period of time and to try and be patient. Having too much pressure can cause bruising or hemorrhaging in the penis. You should never restrict the blood flow to the penis with a device such as a cock ring. Don't be fooled online by fake pictures or pornography about the results you can achieve, you can increase size but only slowly and only by a limited amount.

You need to careful that you select the correct type of penis pump. They can be used to increase the size of the penis, both permanently and temporarily, but some are also designed for those having erectile issues, as the pump can improve the fullness and strength of an erection. Many of the pumps are designed more-or-less solely for help with erectile dysfunction and if you purchase one without adequate research you may disappointed if you don't have any trouble with getting and maintaining an erection.

The things you need to be sure of are that it is has a quick release option, in case you need to end a session quickly, and a pressure gauge so you know you are not overdoing the amount of pressure. You should check that any pump it is the correct size for you (a good pump seller will tell you the size online) and that it has good reviews and comes from a reputable site. Hand pumps are usually the best option as you do not need a great deal of pressure and it is easy to go too far with an electronic pump.

Many advantages come with using penis pumps. It has been shown to make the penis larger with practice and correct usage. Pumps tend not to be costly, they're less risky than other penile enlargement devices, and they don't require insertion into the penis or surgery. Penis pumps can be combined with other methods of penile enlargement such as jelqing and dieting to maximize its effects. If you have health issues such as diabetes, the penis pump may conflict with some of the medication you are taking or make certain symptoms worse.

When choosing the right penis pump, you need to look at many factors. Cost, size, how much you intend to use it, comfort, and figuring out whether you want manual or automatic.

One brand that has been popularized among those serious about really increasing the size of their penis the Hydromax Bathmate series. The beauty of this product is that it comes in several different sizes and three different colors, it is also one of the higher quality builds on the market. Choose between the Bathmate Hercules and the Bathmate Goliath to purchase.

The Bathmate Hercules is a popular model used by thousands of men in over 70 countries. Unlike the typical hand or electronic air pump the Bathmate actually uses water to create the vacuum. It is the original patented Hydro pump globally promoted and used. It is constructed to work while you take a bath or shower using the amazing, satisfying power of water! It lengthens, thickens, strengthens and increases sexual satisfaction for the man looking to improve his penis for himself and his partner(s). It not only works physically, but mentally because it increases one's self-esteem and total confidence.

To use a hydropump you first need to take a warm bath for several minutes to get the blood flowing into your penis and then you fill the pump with water and place it over the penis, pulling it close to the pelvis. Pulling it closer creates more suction and more pressure. Many people find this a much more enjoyable way to use a penis pump. The only thing you need to be careful of is that the water is not too hot or that it is not used for too long as hot water and high pressure can cause blisters if you are not careful.

If you are looking for something a bit bigger, as in thirty percent bigger, then check out the Bathmate Goliath. The largest Hydro pump in the world, the Bathmate Goliath is perfect for men who have larger members than average. Men who have larger penises and male porn actors who are looking for "a boost" can find the maintenance and effectiveness in this device. Easy to use, safe, and can be purchased anywhere in the world. If you aren't please with the product, you have less than two months to return and get a refund guaranteed.

It is suggested to pump once a day, or every other day for 15 to 20 minutes. By doing this regularly, you are keeping your penis healthy and increase the chances of more permanent results. Penis pumps are great to use as long as you know the risks such as pain and discomfort and discoloration. In those cases, it is best to wait and heal before resuming.

There are more drastic versions of penis pumps that some may choose to have implanted into their penis directly. These are more for those struggling with erectile dysfunction but some of the same principles may apply. You can have cylinders places in the erect penis that can be pumped up with a saline fluid to create a harder erection. There is also the option of a metal rod placed in the erection chamber which gives you a very artificially erect penis that may then become difficult to put back away. This last option is really only for those with penises damaged during an accident or surgery.

CHAPTER 10: WHAT IS PENIS STRETCHING?

Penis stretching may be the oldest form of penile enlargement exercises. Many exercises in the advanced stages of penile enlargement training focuses on stretching or bending the penis. It is suggested to first grip the shaft of the penis, right behind the glans. Next, the person is to stretch as hard as they can, but not enough to cause pain, from different directions. Left, right, upwards, and straight forward (horizontal).

When doing these stretches, you should start off slowly and carefully build intensity when necessary. You should not feel any pain. If you do experience any pain or discomfort, then you should stop the exercise immediately. The best way to know if you are stretching correctly is if you feel a sense of tingling, itching, or fatigue. Some men claim they feel a burning sensation, similar to when you are working out at the gym.

Here are a few tips before you begin your penis stretching workout:

1. Work Comfortably: If you feel more comfortable stretching sitting down than standing up, then it is perfectly fine! Whether you are standing or sitting, what is most important is your level of comfort.
2. Start Flat: Before you start stretching while having an erection, you should begin stretching while flaccid (not erect). The first 3 to 6 months should focus on stretching while not having an erection. Once you are more experienced, then you may stretch your erect penis.

3. Healing Time: Give yourself time to heal. Jelqing and stretching can cause red dots, which are normal. However, if much larger discolorations form, you should allow your penis to heal for 48 to 72 hours. This happens when you do not warm up correctly or stretched too hard.
4. Hands versus Aide: You can use your bare hands or have an aide to help you with your stretching. Fabric, rubber gloves, or even baby powder can do the trick.
5. Read before Performing: Don't just jump into stretching. It is a process that takes patience and research, so be sure to read beforehand before beginning your journey to optimum penile growth.

If you feel more comfortable using a penis stretching device, there are several products available to the public. Usually, the product will be called a penis extender or penis stretcher and will increase the penis size in a quick pace. This depends on several factors such as the brand and quality of the device, the time duration of using the device, and if you are incorporating any other physical activity to enlarge your penis. Be sure to research before purchasing.

CHAPTER 11: HOW TO SCHEDULE WORKOUT ROUTINE

Your workout routine will be based on your skill level. Skill levels will usually be divided into three categories: newcomer, beginner, and advanced. Newcomers have no experience in penile enlargement exercises and are just starting out. Beginners are those who have been working out regularly for 2 to 6 months, and advanced individuals are those who have been doing high intensity workouts for 6 or more months. This section will show what newcomers may perform for a schedule workout routine.

The best time to work out is either in the early morning or at night when you are in bed. Many men also suggest exercising in the shower. That is the beauty of jelqing since it takes little to no equipment and can be performed while simultaneously completing other tasks.

Newcomers start off with a conditioning program for the first eight weeks of your training. It mainly focuses on shape, but it works on length and girth as well. This conditioning program has been created for those new to penile enlargement. It helps the penis to slowly and carefully get used to the stresses of exercising. This is vital as the first few weeks of penile enlargement are when the majority of injuries occur. This happens usually because of pushing too far, and too quick. The workouts should be a challenge, but not likely to hurt you. This is only a sample, you can create your own workout program

The first day, you will measure the size of your penis with a tape measure from length and width. This will be done when the penis is flaccid and then erect. The same will be done at the end of each week up to the last day of the program (day 56).

This is a sample of a conditioning workout if you are a beginner:

- Hot Wrap 1x1 rep, 2 minutes
- Hot Kegel Clench 1x60 reps, 3 sec. each
- Basic Stretch 1x5 reps, 30 sec. each
- Helicopter Shake 1x1 rep, 30 sec.
- Wet Jelq 1x80 reps, 3 sec. each
- Helicopter Shake 1x1, 30 sec.
- Hot Kegel Clench: 1x120 reps, 1 sec. each

For the hot wrap, do it for one set and one repetition for two minutes. For the kegel clench exercise, it will be performed twice--once in the beginning and once towards the end of the workout for one set. The first set (beginning of the workout) for 60 reps, three seconds each rep. Double the reps to 120 repetitions for the second time at the end of your workout, only each rep is for one second. The helicopter shake, which is performed twice, is the same number of reps and seconds.

When you feel ready, feel free to add more reps until the eight-week program has been complete. Again, remember to take your time and if you feel discomfort, take small breaks. Here is a second sample program that anyone in the more experienced levels can use to increase length:

- Basic Stretch 2 x 5 40 sec. each
- Helicopter Shake 1 x 1 rep, 30 seconds
- Rotation Stretch 2 x 3 reps, 15 sec. each
- Helicopter Shake 1 x 1 rep, 30 seconds
- Wet Jelq 1 x 170 reps, 3 sec. each
- Hot Kegel Clench 1 x 100 reps, 3 sec. each

It should take roughly 20 minutes to complete. It's best to do these exercises every other day. On your rest day, you can simply get some rest, play, or go shopping to keep your mind busy until the next workout routine.

CHAPTER 12: VIAGRA AND OTHER PILLS, POTIONS AND CREAMS

We've all heard of Viagra and have a good idea of what it is, but the real question is whether it will enlarge your penis. Obviously in one sense the answer is: very much so as the pill allows you to achieve a fuller and longer erection. The question you really want answered is whether that erection will be bigger than your typical erection.

In a physical sense Viagra cannot make your penis increase in weight or volume, it's not a pill that is full of growth hormones or magical flesh extending powers. But the truth is that not all erections are created equally, as you probably full well know, and being able to achieve a fully engorged and powerful erection short term should allow your penis to create more of an imposition in a room and fill you with confidence.

For some people being able to show off their manhood at its peaks might make up for some of the insecurity they have about their penis length. Many will find that just having the extra bulk and stiffness of a full erection is enough to impress any of their partners and will convince them you are a next level lover. It's also true that if you don't achieve a full-blooded erection any increase in length you otherwise achieve will risk going unnoticed in the bedroom.

So how does Viagra actually work? Your nervous system is as active in your penis as anywhere else in your body and when you are sexually stimulated it releases a series of chemicals and enzymes that relax the muscles in your penis, which allows the arteries in your penis to swell up and allows blood to entire the erectile tissue of your penis. All of this inflating and swelling results in an erection which goes away once the sexual stimulation ends.

Viagra simply regulates the enzyme that allows the muscles in the penis to relax so you are able to achieve longer and fuller erections. Contrary to what a lot of films will tell you, giving someone Viagra doesn't cause them to be taken over by an uncontrollable erection: you still need to become aroused to get an erection. It usually takes between thirty minutes to an hour to fully take effect.

If you don't feel that you have any issues getting fully erect then there is not likely too much that Viagra can offer you. Viagra is generally considered a safe drug to use on a regular basis and the side effects are no more scary or frequent than you'd see for a lot of commonly used pills. In some jurisdictions you can even buy it without a prescription. The main concern is for those with already existing conditions or on other medication as it can interfere with other drugs you take and it does lower your blood pressure. Always consult a doctor before using any new drug to be sure you are safe.

The main problem with Viagra is that buying the brand Viagra, which is the market name for Sildenafil, can be quite expensive: especially if you want to use it a lot. You might see some vending machines selling a mysterious blue pill with dubious effects, and you might want to take a chance those will work, but you can instead just buy 'off-brand' versions of Viagra that will be much cheaper and will work. The most common is Kamagra or buying the pill under the name Sildenafil, but you might also want to try Cialis, Spedra, or Levitra. Knock-off versions of Viagra are common outside of the Western world so be careful if you plan to buy online from somewhere like Mexico. Often these won't be as dangerous as much as they are ineffective.

Other options

There are many other proven options for treating erectile dysfunction, one of the more extreme is what is called Prostaglandin E1. Which is an injection that works quickly and very effectively, but it's still an injection. A similar drug also comes in the form of a suppository for the urethra (yes, it is that unpleasant), or as a cream called Alprostadil.

But, what about pills that claim to actually increase penis length? In general you need to be careful with anything that suggests it will do this because realistically what mechanism could you administer chemically that would know to make your penis, and nothing else, grow while not giving you some form of penile cancer?

You might find that general workout enhancement drugs could help in addition to general exercises to either speed or strengthen the process, but there is no guarantee that it would dramatically improve or speed-up the results that consistent exercise will do on its own. It's also quite an expensive route. Certain hormone replacements might help virility and muscle growth, but it isn't something you can undertake safely without proper medical counseling.

When it comes to penis growing pills and creams the market is saturated with choices, which is usually a sign that no one serious has come along yet to dominate it with something that really works well. Perhaps the most common male enhancement supplement is VigRX. The purported effects are a veracious sexual appetite, terrifying hardness of erections, endless supplies of strong and virile sperm, penis growth of anywhere from one to six inches, and an overwhelming sense of having just been ripped-off.

Other brands include Vimax, Pro Solution Pill, Maxirex, Natural Gain Plus, ZyGain, and, a personal favorite, Sir Maximus. How do they claim to work to stimulate human penis growth beyond natural and normal penis size using merely the body's own systems? Well, it's never very clear what the active ingredients are or how they would ultimately do anything to the body that creates growth of the penis. Some sources claim that it increases blood flow to the penis, much like Viagra, which apparently makes the erection longer and that causes a permanently longer penis. Although if that worked you'd possibly expect your penis to look like a deflated balloon the next day. Others claim to be natural sources of testosterone which is not a proven way to increase penis length. They also tend to be the only drugs in the entire world that have no side effects.

Typically they contain various types of herbal solutions or staples of Chinese medicine. If they're not just random concoctions they will be herbs or spices that are traditional or folk aphrodisiacs, some of the most common ingredients being Maca and horny goat weed. Some of these ingredients do have proven efficacy in treating erectile dysfunction and work in a manner similar to Viagra. You will also find that they might include common health supplements like ginseng. If you're lucky the pill might pep you up a bit and give you a stronger erection. Some will also find that the simple placebo effect of taking the pills will change their perception of how long they feel (although not to what the tape measure says).

If you are still interested in supplements then look at what is in the pill you are interested in buying. A lot of the ingredients can be bought separately for mere pennies and will imbue the same positive effects as the pill would and since they are fairly innocuous you could buy an entire bag online and sprinkle them on your breakfast cereal each morning.

Creams might seem like a better option, after all, there are creams for helping to heal skin that is burned or damaged, and by applying cream to the penis itself would in theory allow you to target specific areas of the body for growth. Brands include Revival for Men, Englargo Development Cream, and Swole Cream. Unfortunately the creams often have the same unlikely claims as the pills when it comes to growth. Many will tell you how the cream will seep into the Corpus Cavernosum, the fancy Latin word for the spongy tissue that gets erect, which increases blood flow and somehow permanently makes the penis bigger.

The ingredients are typically a little less useful than those contained in the pills; some will include things like emu oil which is really only a step away from selling you actual snake oil. Some appear to have no active ingredients. With claims that these creams are naturally you'd expect to see coconut oil or beeswax in the ingredients but instead they are synthetic compounds. The penis is a sensitive place; avoid putting suspicious creams on it.

Two options that should have some effectiveness but are not quite surgery are collagen or plasma implants. With the collagen option you are given several injections, or non-needle injections, that place collagen (which is essentially just the same as the yellow fat on your body) under the skin of your penis. They claim this stimulates the body to keep growing collagen in the same area, though undertakers of a similar procedure claim that sometimes it does not remain in the penis and you might end up with a lumpy effect.

With the plasma option, your own blood cells used for healing, platelets, or plasma is injected into specific areas of the penis, which is claimed to simulate re-growth in the region. It is difficult to find too many people who claim to have had these procedures done, but there is more room for these to work, although they would be expensive. It's not clear they would make the penis longer rather than fatter however, or that they would genuinely provide a long-term increase in size.

CHAPTER 13: SURGERY

Exercise, workout routines, jelqing and some of the apparatus on the market can have genuine penis lengthening success, but they do require discipline if they are to work effectively and long term. Surgery is the one option that has proven success and can work fairly quickly although some options do still require you to use weights after surgery to stretch the penis out.

The catch is that it is expensive and not always safe or recommended. Many of the more extreme operations cannot be legally done in the West and going abroad to have the ligaments in your penis stretch out is not always the best idea to nurture. It is, nevertheless, still an option that some people wish to try out or explore.

For some men surgery is a more vital option if they have an abnormally small or disfigured penis and they want to gain basic use out of if it and it is generally for these men that the procedures are carried out. The main three types of surgery you will get are penis lengthening, penis widening, or a scrotum lift.

With lengthening the ligament, the tissue connecting different parts of the body, between the pubic bone and the top of the penis is cut which makes the penis drop forward, usually by one or two inches. The ligament is then re-attached lower down and given a skin graft to heal.

Widening usually uses a form of fat transfer, or liposuction, and is down without incision into the shaft of the penis. You can also AlloDerm regenerative tissue under the penis which is more expensive but has more consistent results. Finally the scrotum can be given a general lift if it is felt to be too saggy, or the webbing penis the penis and scrotum can be cut to reduce any bunching up that might be making the penis appear to be smaller.

There is a risk with these surgeries that you will not be happy with the actual results, appearance is just as important as length, and some doctors will not happily perform them on a 'normal' looking penis. The cost can be $3000 to $10,000 which some may feel is a lot of money, or, if you worry a lot about your penis, a small amount of a happier life. Only you can decide if surgery is for you. You should use the best surgeon you can find and are happy to pay for. Never settle for quick and cheap results with someone you do not trust and avoid surgery unless you have a reason to believe your life is significantly hampered by the length of your penis.

CHAPTER 14: PENIS EXTENDERS

Nearly all of the main methods of penis extension have been covered so far in this book, but the world of penis extension tools is a large and colorful one, so here we will cover some of the less known tools and options you have.

One of the most obvious, and perhaps rightfully overlooked, ways of extending your penis is to simply get a prosthetic extender made of silicone or another malleable material to place on the end of your penis during sex. Clearly this would reduce stimulation and it might not look ideal, however if you find your concern about your penis is merely that it is not long enough to pleasure a woman this might just address your concerns.

There are many of these sold as little more than gags but the transvestite community has a large range that have been designed for both comfort and dignity. They are not always the cheapest option, but it is a pain free and ultimately instant fix. Some devices bought from sex shops are built to give you extra stimulation and can make sex fun or enhance the appearance of your penis. They are simply attached and can come in a variety of colors or they can even be translucent if you prefer.

To actually extend the penis you have there are many penis extenders and penis stretchers on the market that are available for you to buy. Most of these are about as complicated as they sound – they are devices for literally stretching the penis with the intention for it to grow longer. The logic is that it will cause tearing in the way that working out tears up muscles that will then be healed back stronger and longer than before.

The devices vary in how they work and operate and even their intention. Some of them are made for fixing issues with the curvature of the penis but many are built to actually stretch the penis. The base of the penis has a ring placed around it and then the tip is placed in a small carrier. The ring and base are connected by a metal rod which is then little by little extended with the intention to stretch the skin. Other, more basic devices are more like a piece of elastic that you place around the penis and pull forwards.

Clearly this will stretch the skin of the penis but whether all it will do is stretch the skin out beyond the actual shaft of the penis is not entirely clear. If you are intended to use one make sure you find one that is solidly built and try to use it in conjunction with other penis growing methods. There is good evidence that using certain extenders such as the Andropenis for several hours a day over several months could help improve penis length. This is quite a big commitment however.

Another penis extending machine is the electric shock ring expander. Most of the devices appear to come with Chinese text on them and have no English language equivalent. Quite simply you attach 4 or 5 rings along the shaft of your penis and they are then exposed to a series of electric shocks. These shocks are supposed to make the penis contract and then relax which is meant to relax muscles and fill the penis with blood. The principle sounds similar to many of the other penis enlarging devices but it's not clear the shocks would work to do this and it is not the most popular product out there. Chances are you might just end up with a slightly fried penis.

Penis hanging or penis weights use a similar principle to the penis extenders by using tearing and stretching to try and induce increased length. Essentially they are just devises for attaching a weight to the penis and then letting gravity to a do the work of stretching it. Typically they are like small rings that are placed just before the glands and weighed down with a metal ball.

The plus of the weights is that they are not always that expensive and they should not take too long to use every day, not is there too much effort required of you. Similar techniques have been used successfully by those trying to re-grow their foreskins for many years now and it might interest you to research the movement and to take lessons here.

You should be cautious though as stretching your penis with weights could cause damage: if you do decide to try it make sure you are comfortable with it every step of the way and try to limit the time you use it to no more than 10-20 minutes a session. Generally speaking the penis extenders or stretchers without using weights will be safer and more comfortable.

CHAPTER 15: SAFETY AND OTHER HELPFUL TIPS

The best way to conclude this booklet is by discussing the importance of safety. While there are plenty advantages of using these penile enlargement techniques, it is important to go over the risks that you may or may not encounter. This way, you are prepared and will know what to do if an accident occurs.

1. Never jelq with a full erection. Partial erections are okay, but to avoid injury it is best to not be 100% erect. Anywhere below 80% is ideal.

2. With any exercise, do not begin at the top of the glans (head). Many of these exercises will begin at the base of the penis, closest to your pelvis.

3. Take your time when performing these exercises. You aren't supposed to yank until you feel pain or go over the time limit for each rep. It isn't a race; as the saying goes, patience is a virtue.

4. Always warm up. When you go to the gym, you warm up with a few light reps or perform some stretches. The same applies with penile enlargement exercises. Whether you are a newbie or an advanced learner, you must always warm up to increase blow flow. Use a warm towel or a towel dipped in warm water and wrap it around the shaft.

5. Always use the OK style grip. Whether it is the standard (palms up) or overhand (palms down), it is important to know how to restrict blood flow when needed.

6. Consistency is key. The grip should be the same throughout each exercise. It's easy enough to go against the pattern you have been using as you grip the penis.

7. A tube of lube helps--really. Buy a bottle of water-based lubricant such as Astroglide to make to avoid chafing and discomfort. Plus, it is easier to wash off than oil-based lubes. If you use an oil-based lubricant, keep in mind you are increasing the risk for infection.

Now that you know the list of safety precautions and proper ways to handle certain situations, you can begin your training for a new and improved penis!

CONCLUSION

Now you have a basic understand of penis enlargement and what you can do to make significant changes in your life. You should know the anatomy of the penis, how sex hormones play a role in the body, how diet affects growth and libido, and exercises that promote shape, length, and girth.

Hopefully these tips will be useful to you as you begin your journey to thicker, longer, and stronger erections. Penile enlargement is a serious goal to follow and by researching and putting together a daily routine, you can find positive changes appearing in no time. Each step is a milestone closer to your goal; it takes patience and dedication to get what you want.

If you are still self-conscious about the size of your penis after having success with extra length then consider using therapy or hypnotherapy to become more accepting of the length and strength of your penis. There is evidence that some reassurance from a healthcare professional can make your more comfortable and accepting of the size you have achieved. You might consider taking a break from consuming too much pornography or to try and change your typical viewing habits. There can be a lot of fun and self-satisfaction in trying to look like a porn star, but don't forget that male porn stars are chosen specifically for their large penises.

In addition you could turn to penis exercising groups: found online and in larger cities. This works as a kind of support group to help you reach your goals but also think of these people as gym buddies that will push you to go further and to remind you of the achievements you can make if you stick with your routines.

How you use your penis is just as important at how big it is in terms of pleasuring a woman so don't overlook techniques for pleasuring her and making yourself feel and appear sexier. It is little use having a larger penis if you still can't use it properly and you should make sure that any erection you achieve is as full and hard as it can be. Take your time with love making and become focused so that you learn how to become fully aroused.

Remember to be confident in yourself. Whether you grow two inches or none at all, keep in mind that all bodies are beautiful. Everyone has insecurities over one or more body parts/areas, so it helps to know you aren't alone. Good luck on your journey to penis enlargement success!